Crohn's Disease Cookbook

A Culinary Journey to Manage Crohn's Disease

Lisa Hultin

Copyright

No part of this book should be copied, reproduced without the author's permission © 2024

TABLE OF CONTENT

Part I. Understanding Crohn's Disease

Overview of Crohn's Disease

Crohn's disease is a chronic inflammatory bowel condition that significantly impacts the gastrointestinal tract. Characterized by inflammation of the digestive system, Crohn's can affect any part of the digestive tract, from the mouth to the anus. This inflammatory process often leads to a range of symptoms, including abdominal pain, diarrhea, fatigue, and weight loss. Crohn's disease is classified as an autoimmune disorder, wherein the immune system mistakenly attacks healthy cells in the digestive tract, triggering inflammation.

The exact cause of Crohn's disease remains unclear, but a combination of genetic, environmental, and immune system factors is believed to contribute to its development. While the condition can manifest at any age, it commonly appears in individuals between the ages of 15 and 35. Crohn's disease is a chronic condition, meaning that it persists over an extended period and may involve periods of remission and flare-ups.

The impact of Crohn's disease extends beyond physical symptoms, affecting the overall quality of life of those diagnosed. Managing the condition involves a multifaceted approach, including medication, lifestyle modifications, and dietary adjustments. Individuals with Crohn's often require ongoing medical monitoring and collaboration with healthcare professionals to tailor treatment plans to their unique needs. Understanding and addressing the challenges posed by Crohn's disease is essential for both patients and healthcare providers in fostering effective management strategies and improving the overall well-being of those living with this chronic inflammatory condition.

Historical Background

The historical background of Crohn's disease dates back to the early 20th century when it was first recognized as a distinct medical condition. In 1932, Dr.

Burrill B. Crohn, Dr. Leon Ginzburg, and Dr. Gordon D. Oppenheimer identified and documented a series of cases with similar inflammatory bowel symptoms. Their seminal work, published in the Journal of the American Medical Association, marked the formal recognition of what would later be known as Crohn's disease.

Initially termed "terminal ileitis," the researchers soon realized that the condition could affect various parts of the gastrointestinal tract. They subsequently named it Crohn's disease in honor of Dr. Burrill B. Crohn, acknowledging his significant contributions to its understanding. Over the following decades, medical advancements and technological developments, such as endoscopy and imaging techniques, enhanced the ability to diagnose and study the disease.

Crohn's disease has evolved from an enigmatic gastrointestinal disorder to a well-recognized chronic condition affecting millions worldwide. Ongoing research and medical progress continue to deepen our understanding of its complex etiology, paving the way for improved diagnostic methods and targeted therapies. The historical journey of Crohn's disease reflects the collaborative efforts of medical pioneers, highlighting the ongoing commitment to unraveling the intricacies of this inflammatory bowel disorder for the benefit of those affected.

Understanding Inflammatory Bowel Disease (IBD)

Inflammatory Bowel Disease (IBD) comprises a group of chronic disorders characterized by inflammation of the gastrointestinal tract, primarily including Crohn's disease and ulcerative colitis. Unlike temporary gastrointestinal issues, IBD involves persistent and often unpredictable inflammation that can affect various parts of the digestive system.

The exact cause of IBD remains elusive, but it is believed to result from a complex interplay of genetic, environmental, and immune system factors. The immune system, misinterpreting normal gut bacteria or food as threats, triggers an inflammatory response, leading to symptoms like abdominal pain, diarrhea, weight loss, and fatigue.

Crohn's disease can affect any part of the digestive tract, from the mouth to the anus, causing deep-seated inflammation, while ulcerative colitis primarily impacts the colon and rectum, resulting in continuous inflammation along the mucosal lining.

Managing IBD involves a personalized approach, often combining medications to suppress inflammation, lifestyle modifications, and, in some cases, surgery. The impact of IBD extends beyond physical symptoms, influencing mental health and overall quality of life. Regular monitoring and collaboration with healthcare professionals are crucial for effective disease management and improving the well-being of those living with IBD. Ongoing research continues to uncover new insights into the complexities of IBD, offering hope for better treatments and an improved understanding of this chronic inflammatory condition.

Chapter One

Nutritional Requirements for

Crohn's Patients

Nutritional requirements for individuals with Crohn's disease are critical for managing symptoms, supporting overall health, and preventing nutrient deficiencies. Due to the inflammatory nature of the condition and potential challenges in nutrient absorption, specific considerations must be taken into account:

1. Protein Intake: Protein is essential for tissue repair and overall health. Including lean meats, fish, eggs, and plant-based sources like tofu and legumes can help maintain muscle mass and support healing.

2. Caloric Needs: During active disease or flare-ups, individuals with Crohn's may experience increased energy expenditure. Consuming an adequate number of calories from a variety of sources helps prevent malnutrition and supports energy levels.

3. Vitamins and Minerals: Due to potential malabsorption, monitoring vitamin and mineral levels is crucial. Vitamin D, calcium, iron, and B vitamins are commonly affected. Dietary sources and supplements may be recommended based on individual needs.

4. Hydration: Chronic diarrhea and inflammation can lead to dehydration. Staying well-hydrated is essential for maintaining electrolyte balance and supporting digestive function.

5. Fiber Management: While a high-fiber diet is generally encouraged for digestive health, individuals with Crohn's may need to limit fiber during flare-ups. Gradual reintroduction of soluble fiber from well-cooked fruits and vegetables may be considered during remission.

6. Omega-3 Fatty Acids: Foods rich in omega-3 fatty acids, such as fatty fish, flaxseeds, and walnuts, can have anti-inflammatory effects and support heart health.

7. Probiotics: Incorporating probiotic-rich foods like yogurt or taking supplements may help maintain a healthy balance of gut bacteria, promoting overall digestive health.

8. Individualized Diet Plans: Working with a registered dietitian or healthcare professional is crucial for tailoring nutritional strategies to individual needs. Personalized diet plans can address specific triggers and preferences.

Regular monitoring of nutritional status through blood tests and professional guidance ensures that individuals with Crohn's disease can adapt their diets to manage symptoms, promote healing, and maintain optimal health. It's important to consider the dynamic nature of the disease, adjusting dietary strategies based on individual responses and disease activity.

Addressing Nutrient Deficiencies

Addressing nutrient deficiencies is a critical aspect of managing Crohn's disease, a condition that often leads to malabsorption and increased nutrient requirements. Here are key considerations for addressing nutrient deficiencies in individuals with Crohn's:

1. Regular Monitoring: Regular blood tests and nutritional assessments help identify specific deficiencies. Monitoring levels of vitamins (such as B12, D, and folate), minerals (like iron and calcium), and

other essential nutrients provides a baseline for intervention.

2. Supplementation: In cases of identified deficiencies, targeted supplementation may be recommended. This can involve oral supplements or, in severe cases, intravenous administration to ensure optimal nutrient levels.

3. Dietary Modifications: Tailoring the diet to include nutrient-dense foods is crucial. Incorporating a variety of fruits, vegetables, lean proteins, and whole grains can help meet nutritional needs. Adjusting the diet to address specific deficiencies, such as increasing iron-rich foods for anemia, is common.

4. Individualized Plans: Working with a registered dietitian or healthcare professional ensures a personalized approach to addressing nutrient deficiencies. They can develop a dietary plan that considers the individual's preferences, triggers, and specific nutritional requirements.

5. Incorporating Easily Absorbed Forms: Choosing foods and supplements with easily absorbed forms of nutrients can enhance absorption. For instance, selecting heme iron from animal sources or vitamin D3 instead of D2 can be more effective.

6. Probiotics: Introducing probiotics may enhance nutrient absorption by promoting a healthy balance of gut bacteria. Probiotics can support gut health, potentially improving the absorption of certain nutrients.

7. Monitoring Medications: Some medications prescribed for Crohn's disease may affect nutrient absorption. Close monitoring and adjustments to the diet or supplementation can help counteract potential deficiencies associated with these medications.

Addressing nutrient deficiencies in Crohn's disease requires a comprehensive and multifaceted approach. Regular collaboration with healthcare professionals ensures ongoing monitoring and adjustment of dietary and supplementation strategies, ultimately contributing to improved nutritional status and overall well-being.

Identifying and Avoiding Dietary Triggers

Identifying and avoiding dietary triggers is crucial for managing Crohn's disease, as certain foods can exacerbate inflammation and contribute to symptom flare-ups. Here are key strategies for recognizing and steering clear of potential triggers:

1. Keep a Food Diary: Recording daily food intake helps identify patterns between specific foods and symptom exacerbation. Documenting meals, snacks, and symptom occurrences assists in pinpointing potential triggers.

2. Gradual Introduction of Foods: After a period of symptom management, gradually reintroduce eliminated foods to observe their impact. This cautious approach helps identify individual tolerances and sensitivities.

3. Common Trigger Foods: Certain foods are known to be common triggers for individuals with Crohn's. These include spicy foods, high-fiber items, dairy, caffeine, and certain fats. Identifying and limiting intake of these triggers can be beneficial.

4. Monitor Symptoms: Regularly monitor Crohn's symptoms, such as abdominal pain, diarrhea, and fatigue. Connecting symptom patterns with specific foods provides valuable insights into trigger identification.

5. Consult with a Dietitian: Collaborate with a registered dietitian or healthcare professional specializing in inflammatory bowel diseases. Their expertise can guide you in creating an individualized

diet plan tailored to your specific triggers and nutritional needs.

6. Elimination Diet: Consider an elimination diet under the guidance of a healthcare professional. This involves systematically removing potential trigger foods and reintroducing them to assess their impact on symptoms.

7. Consideration of Non-Food Triggers: Beyond dietary factors, non-food triggers such as stress, medications, and hormonal changes can influence Crohn's symptoms. Holistic management includes addressing these aspects for comprehensive care.

8. Stay Informed: Keep up-to-date with current research and medical advice regarding dietary recommendations for Crohn's disease. This ensures that you are equipped with the latest information to make informed decisions about your diet.

Identifying and avoiding dietary triggers requires a personalized and patient-centered approach. Through careful observation, collaboration with healthcare professionals, and a proactive stance towards nutrition, individuals with Crohn's can optimize their dietary choices to manage symptoms and enhance their quality of life.

Common Triggers

Common triggers in the diet of individuals with Crohn's disease can significantly influence the course of the condition. Understanding and managing these triggers is crucial for symptom control and overall well-being:

1. High-Fiber Foods: Insoluble fiber, found in seeds, nuts, and rough vegetables, can be challenging to digest and may aggravate symptoms. Opting for cooked, peeled, or finely chopped versions of fruits and vegetables can make them more manageable.

2. Spicy Foods: Spices and hot peppers can irritate the digestive tract, leading to increased inflammation and discomfort. Minimizing or avoiding spicy foods may help alleviate symptoms.

3. Dairy Products: Lactose intolerance is common in individuals with Crohn's disease, as inflammation can affect the production of lactase. Choosing lactose-free alternatives or incorporating probiotic-rich dairy may be better tolerated.

4. Caffeine and Alcohol: Both caffeine and alcohol can be irritants to the gastrointestinal tract, potentially

triggering inflammation. Limiting or avoiding these substances may help manage symptoms.

5. Certain Fats: High-fat foods, especially those rich in saturated and trans fats, can be challenging for individuals with Crohn's to digest. Choosing healthier fats from sources like olive oil and fatty fish may be more tolerable.

6. Raw Fruits and Vegetables: The tough fibers in raw fruits and vegetables can be harsh on the digestive system. Cooking or peeling these foods can make them easier to digest while retaining nutritional benefits.

7. Processed and Fried Foods: Highly processed foods and fried items often contain additives and unhealthy fats that may contribute to inflammation. Opting for whole, minimally processed foods can be a healthier choice.

8. Carbonated Beverages: Carbonated drinks can contribute to gas and bloating, which may exacerbate symptoms in individuals with Crohn's. Choosing still beverages and staying well-hydrated with water is advisable.

Individual responses to these triggers vary, making it crucial for individuals with Crohn's to maintain a food diary and work closely with healthcare professionals, including dietitians, to identify and manage specific dietary triggers. Tailoring the diet to individual tolerances helps minimize symptom flare-ups and optimize nutritional intake.

Personalized Trigger Management

Personalized trigger management is a cornerstone of effective Crohn's disease care, recognizing the unique responses individuals have to specific dietary and lifestyle factors. Here are key elements in creating a personalized approach to trigger management:

1. Food Diary: Keeping a detailed food diary allows individuals to track their daily food intake, symptoms, and any correlations between specific foods and symptom exacerbation. This observational tool is crucial for identifying personalized triggers.

2. Gradual Reintroduction: After a period of symptom management, gradually reintroducing eliminated foods one at a time helps pinpoint specific triggers. This gradual approach, under the guidance of healthcare professionals, allows for a more accurate assessment of tolerances.

3. Individualized Elimination Diets: Tailoring elimination diets to an individual's specific symptoms and dietary history can be beneficial. Eliminating potential trigger foods and reintroducing them systematically helps identify problematic items.

4. Consultation with Healthcare Professionals: Working closely with a healthcare team, including a registered dietitian and gastroenterologist, ensures a comprehensive and personalized approach. Professionals can provide guidance, interpret symptom patterns, and recommend dietary modifications.

5. Consideration of Non-Food Triggers: Beyond dietary factors, non-food triggers such as stress, medications, and hormonal changes play a role in Crohn's disease. Personalized management involves addressing these aspects alongside dietary considerations.

6. Genetic and Gut Microbiome Factors: Emerging research suggests that genetic factors and variations in the gut microbiome contribute to individual responses to specific foods. Understanding these factors can inform a more targeted approach to trigger management.

7. Ongoing Monitoring: Crohn's disease is dynamic, and triggers may change over time. Regular monitoring of symptoms, dietary responses, and overall well-being

allows for adjustments in trigger management strategies.

By embracing a personalized trigger management approach, individuals with Crohn's can gain greater control over their symptoms, enhance their quality of life, and optimize their nutritional intake. This tailored strategy empowers individuals to make informed choices that align with their unique physiological responses, fostering a proactive and sustainable approach to managing Crohn's disease.

Chapter Two

The Importance of a Balanced Diet

A balanced diet is of paramount importance for overall health and well-being, and it holds particular significance for individuals managing conditions like Crohn's disease. Here's why maintaining a balanced diet is crucial:

1. Nutrient Supply: A balanced diet provides a diverse array of essential nutrients, including vitamins, minerals, proteins, carbohydrates, and fats. These nutrients are fundamental for supporting bodily functions, promoting tissue repair, and ensuring optimal immune function.

2. Energy and Weight Management: A well-balanced diet supplies the energy needed for daily activities and helps maintain a healthy weight. For individuals with Crohn's disease, achieving and sustaining an

appropriate weight is vital for managing symptoms and promoting overall health.

3. Gut Health: A diet rich in fiber, from sources like fruits, vegetables, and whole grains, promotes a healthy gut microbiome and aids in digestion. For individuals with Crohn's, finding a balance that supports gut health without exacerbating symptoms is crucial.

4. Inflammation Control: Certain foods possess anti-inflammatory properties, contributing to the management of chronic inflammatory conditions like Crohn's disease. Omega-3 fatty acids, found in fatty fish and flaxseeds, are known for their anti-inflammatory effects.

5. Disease Management: A balanced diet is an integral component of disease management, helping individuals better cope with the challenges of chronic conditions. Nutrient-rich foods contribute to improved resilience and an enhanced ability to manage symptoms.

6. Prevention of Nutrient Deficiencies: A balanced diet helps prevent nutrient deficiencies, which are common in individuals with inflammatory bowel diseases like Crohn's. Addressing nutrient deficiencies is crucial for

overall health and can positively impact disease outcomes.

7. Mental Health: Nutrient-dense foods, such as those found in a balanced diet, play a role in supporting mental health. Proper nutrition can positively influence mood, cognitive function, and overall mental well-being.

For those with Crohn's disease, tailoring a balanced diet to individual tolerances and nutritional needs is essential. Collaborating with healthcare professionals, including dietitians and gastroenterologists, helps create a personalized dietary plan that optimally manages symptoms, supports overall health, and enhances the quality of life for individuals navigating the complexities of Crohn's disease.

Incorporating Variety for Nutrient Diversity

Incorporating a diverse range of foods into the diet is essential for nutrient diversity and optimal health, especially for individuals managing conditions like Crohn's disease. Here's why variety matters:

1. Comprehensive Nutrition: Different foods provide distinct arrays of vitamins, minerals, antioxidants, and

phytochemicals. Consuming a variety of foods ensures a comprehensive intake of nutrients, supporting overall health and wellness.

2. Microbiome Health: A diverse diet promotes a healthy gut microbiome, crucial for individuals with Crohn's disease. A rich variety of plant-based foods, whole grains, and fermented products contribute to a balanced gut flora, influencing digestion and immune function.

3. Preventing Nutrient Deficiencies: A varied diet helps prevent nutrient deficiencies, a common concern for those with Crohn's. By incorporating a range of nutrient sources, individuals can better meet their nutritional needs, supporting energy levels and preventing malnutrition.

4. Reducing Food Sensitivities: Consuming a wide range of foods may reduce the likelihood of developing sensitivities or intolerances. A diverse diet helps avoid overreliance on specific foods, mitigating the risk of triggering inflammation or discomfort.

5. Enhancing Flavor and Enjoyment: Variety adds excitement and enjoyment to meals, making it easier to adhere to dietary recommendations. Exploring different flavors, textures, and culinary techniques can

make the eating experience more satisfying for individuals with Crohn's.

6. Managing Dietary Restrictions: For those with specific dietary restrictions due to Crohn's disease, incorporating variety within tolerated food groups becomes even more crucial. It ensures a well-rounded and enjoyable eating experience while adhering to individual tolerances.

7. Catering to Changing Preferences: Dietary needs and preferences can change over time, influenced by symptom management, treatment plans, and lifestyle factors. A diverse diet provides flexibility, allowing individuals to adapt their eating habits to evolving circumstances.

Creating a diverse and well-rounded diet involves including a spectrum of fruits, vegetables, whole grains, lean proteins, and healthy fats. Collaboration with healthcare professionals, especially dietitians, can guide individuals with Crohn's in designing a personalized, varied, and nutrient-rich eating plan that aligns with their specific needs and preferences.

Balancing Macronutrients for Digestive Comfort

Balancing macronutrients—proteins, carbohydrates, and fats—is crucial for individuals with Crohn's disease to promote digestive comfort and overall well-being. Here's why achieving this balance is significant:

1. Protein for Healing and Maintenance: Adequate protein intake is essential for tissue repair and maintenance, crucial for individuals with Crohn's experiencing inflammation. Lean sources such as poultry, fish, tofu, and legumes provide essential amino acids without overburdening the digestive system.

2. Carbohydrates for Energy: Carbohydrates are the body's primary energy source. Choosing easily digestible, complex carbohydrates from sources like rice, oats, and sweet potatoes provides sustained energy without causing digestive distress.

3. Healthy Fats for Nutrient Absorption: Incorporating healthy fats, such as those found in avocados, nuts, and olive oil, supports nutrient absorption and helps maintain a healthy weight. Including moderate

amounts of these fats can enhance the overall nutritional profile of meals.

4. Fiber Management: While fiber is crucial for gut health, individuals with Crohn's often need to manage fiber intake. Choosing soluble fiber sources like oatmeal, bananas, and cooked vegetables can support digestive comfort without exacerbating symptoms.

5. Portion Control for Digestive Ease: Balancing macronutrients involves mindful portion control. Smaller, more frequent meals can ease digestion and prevent overwhelming the gastrointestinal tract, especially during flare-ups.

6. Hydration: Although not a macronutrient, proper hydration is integral for digestive health. It aids in nutrient absorption, softens stool, and prevents dehydration. Water, herbal teas, and broths contribute to overall digestive comfort.

Individualized dietary plans that prioritize a balanced distribution of macronutrients help manage symptoms and support digestive comfort in individuals with Crohn's disease. Collaborating with a registered dietitian or healthcare professional ensures that dietary choices align with specific needs, tolerances, and nutritional requirements for optimal well-being.

Chapter Three

Causes and Risk Factors

The causes and risk factors of Crohn's disease, a chronic inflammatory bowel disorder, are multifaceted and involve a combination of genetic, environmental, and immune system influences. Understanding these factors is crucial for better management and prevention.

Genetic Factors:

Crohn's disease often exhibits a familial clustering, suggesting a genetic predisposition. Individuals with a first-degree relative, such as a parent or sibling, diagnosed with Crohn's have a higher risk of developing the condition. Specific gene mutations, such as those associated with the NOD2 gene, are linked to an increased susceptibility to Crohn's, although not everyone with these mutations develops the disease.

Environmental Factors:

Environmental elements, including lifestyle and external exposures, play a role in triggering or exacerbating Crohn's disease. Factors such as diet, smoking, and microbial infections have been implicated. Dietary habits rich in processed foods, high in fat, and low in fiber may contribute to the development of Crohn's, while certain infections may trigger an abnormal immune response leading to inflammation.

Immune System Dysfunction:

Crohn's disease is classified as an autoimmune disorder, where the immune system mistakenly attacks healthy cells in the digestive tract, leading to chronic inflammation. The exact mechanisms triggering this immune response are not fully understood, but a dysregulated immune system is a central element in the disease pathogenesis.

Risk Factors:

1. Age: While Crohn's disease can develop at any age, it most commonly manifests in individuals between 15 and 35 years old.

2. Ethnicity: Certain ethnic groups, such as Ashkenazi Jews, are at a higher risk of developing Crohn's disease.

3. Geography: People living in urban or industrialized areas have a higher incidence of Crohn's compared to those in rural regions.

4. Smoking: Cigarette smoking is a significant risk factor for Crohn's disease, and it often exacerbates the severity of symptoms.

5. Nonsteroidal Anti-Inflammatory Drugs (NSAIDs): Long-term use of NSAIDs, such as ibuprofen, may increase the risk of developing Crohn's.

6. Appendectomy: Removal of the appendix, especially during early life, may be associated with a decreased risk of developing Crohn's disease.

While these factors contribute to the risk of Crohn's, the interplay between genetics and environmental triggers remains complex. Ongoing research aims to uncover more insights into the intricate mechanisms that lead to Crohn's disease, fostering improved prevention and management strategies for individuals affected by this chronic condition.

Diagnosing Crohn's Disease

Diagnosing Crohn's disease involves a comprehensive approach that combines clinical evaluations, medical imaging, laboratory tests, and sometimes invasive procedures. Due to the complexity of symptoms and the similarities with other gastrointestinal conditions, a thorough diagnostic process is essential.

Clinical Evaluation:

1. Medical History: The healthcare provider will take a detailed medical history, exploring the patient's symptoms, family history of inflammatory bowel disease, and any relevant lifestyle factors.

2. Physical Examination: A thorough physical examination may reveal signs of abdominal tenderness, weight loss, and other symptoms associated with Crohn's disease.

Laboratory Tests:

1. Blood Tests: Blood tests can help identify markers of inflammation, anemia, and nutritional deficiencies. Elevated levels of certain biomarkers, such as C-reactive protein (CRP) and erythrocyte sedimentation rate (ESR), may indicate inflammation in the body.

2. Stool Tests: Analyzing stool samples can provide insights into digestive health, identifying factors such as infections, inflammation, or malabsorption.

Medical Imaging:

1. Endoscopy: Procedures like colonoscopy or sigmoidoscopy involve inserting a flexible tube with a camera into the digestive tract to directly visualize the intestinal lining. This allows for the assessment of inflammation, ulceration, and other abnormalities.

2. Imaging Studies: X-rays, CT scans, and magnetic resonance imaging (MRI) may be utilized to capture detailed images of the digestive tract, helping to identify areas of inflammation, strictures, or fistulas.

Biopsy:

During endoscopic procedures, tissue samples (biopsies) may be collected from the affected areas for microscopic examination. This helps confirm the diagnosis and rule out other gastrointestinal conditions.

Capsule Endoscopy:

In some cases, a patient may swallow a small capsule containing a camera, allowing for visualization of the small intestine, which is challenging to access with traditional endoscopic procedures.

Differential Diagnosis:

Crohn's disease shares symptoms with other gastrointestinal conditions such as ulcerative colitis, irritable bowel syndrome (IBS), and celiac disease. The diagnostic process involves differentiating between these conditions to ensure accurate and targeted treatment.

Diagnosing Crohn's disease is a collaborative effort between healthcare professionals, including gastroenterologists, radiologists, and pathologists. The goal is to establish a clear understanding of the disease's extent, severity, and specific characteristics, allowing for personalized treatment plans to manage symptoms and improve the quality of life for individuals with Crohn's.

Treatment Options

The treatment of Crohn's disease aims to alleviate symptoms, induce and maintain remission, and improve the overall quality of life for individuals affected by this chronic inflammatory condition. Treatment plans are highly individualized, considering the severity of symptoms, the location and extent of inflammation, and the patient's overall health. Several approaches, including medications, lifestyle modifications, and, in some cases, surgery, are employed to manage Crohn's disease effectively.

Medications:

1. Anti-Inflammatory Drugs: Aminosalicylates, such as mesalamine, help control inflammation and are commonly prescribed for mild to moderate cases.

2. Corticosteroids: For more severe inflammation, corticosteroids like prednisone may be used short-term to quickly suppress the immune response and alleviate symptoms. Long-term use is avoided due to potential side effects.

3. Immunomodulators: Medications like azathioprine, methotrexate, and thiopurines work by modulating the immune system, reducing inflammation and preventing disease progression.

4. Biologics: Monoclonal antibodies like infliximab, adalimumab, and vedolizumab target specific pathways involved in inflammation. Biologics are often prescribed for moderate to severe cases and can induce and maintain remission.

5. Antibiotics: In cases with bacterial overgrowth or fistulas, antibiotics like metronidazole or ciprofloxacin may be recommended.

Lifestyle Modifications:

1. Dietary Changes: While no specific diet cures Crohn's disease, some individuals find relief by modifying their diet. Low-residue diets, elimination diets, or specific carbohydrate diets may be explored under the guidance of a healthcare professional.

2. Nutritional Supplements: In cases of malnutrition or nutrient deficiencies, nutritional supplementation, including enteral nutrition or total parenteral nutrition (TPN), may be recommended.

3. Hydration: Maintaining adequate hydration is essential, especially during flare-ups with diarrhea or vomiting, to prevent dehydration and support overall health.

Surgery:

Surgery becomes an option when medications and lifestyle modifications are insufficient or complications arise. Common surgical procedures for Crohn's disease include:
- Strictureplasty: Widening of narrowed areas in the small intestine.
- Bowel Resection: Removal of damaged portions of the digestive tract.
- Fistula Repair: Closing abnormal connections between organs.

Symptom Management:

1. Anti-Diarrheal Medications: Medications like loperamide can help control diarrhea during flare-ups.

2. Pain Management: Analgesics or nonsteroidal anti-inflammatory drugs (NSAIDs) may be used for pain relief, but caution is advised due to the potential for exacerbating symptoms.

Ongoing Monitoring:

Regular follow-up with healthcare professionals is crucial to assess treatment efficacy, monitor for side effects, and make adjustments to the treatment plan as needed. Periodic imaging, blood tests, and endoscopic evaluations may be performed to track disease progression and response to treatment.

The choice of treatment depends on the individual's specific case, and healthcare professionals work closely with patients to tailor a comprehensive and effective plan. It's important for individuals with Crohn's disease to communicate openly with their healthcare team, adhere to prescribed treatments, and make necessary lifestyle adjustments to optimize their overall well-being.

Chapter Four

Importance of Nutrition in Crohn's Management

Nutrition plays a pivotal role in the management of Crohn's disease, a chronic inflammatory bowel condition. Individuals with Crohn's often face challenges such as malabsorption, nutrient deficiencies, and difficulty maintaining a healthy weight due to inflammation and gastrointestinal symptoms. A well-balanced and tailored diet can significantly impact the overall well-being of those living with Crohn's.

Optimal nutrition is crucial for managing symptoms, promoting healing, and preventing complications. In periods of active inflammation or flare-ups, a focus on easily digestible and low-fiber foods can help reduce gastrointestinal distress. Adequate intake of essential nutrients such as protein, vitamins, and minerals becomes imperative to address potential deficiencies.

Tailoring the diet to individual tolerances is key, as triggers can vary among individuals. Some may find relief through a low-residue diet, avoiding foods that are hard to digest, while others may benefit from specific dietary exclusions, such as lactose or gluten.

Consultation with a registered dietitian or healthcare professional is essential to develop a personalized nutrition plan. Additionally, monitoring nutritional status through regular assessments can guide adjustments to the diet or the incorporation of nutritional supplements when necessary. Overall, a well-managed and nutrient-rich diet is integral to enhancing the quality of life and supporting the overall health of individuals navigating the complexities of Crohn's disease.

Tips for Meal Planning and Preparation

Meal planning and preparation are essential components of managing Crohn's disease, aiming to provide nutrient-rich, easily digestible, and enjoyable meals while minimizing gastrointestinal distress. Here are key tips to consider:

1. Diversify Your Diet: Include a variety of foods to ensure a broad spectrum of nutrients. This can help

manage potential nutrient deficiencies and provide a more enjoyable eating experience.

2. Portion Control: Smaller, more frequent meals can be gentler on the digestive system. Consider dividing daily food intake into several smaller portions to help manage symptoms and prevent discomfort.

3. Hydration is Key: Staying well-hydrated is crucial for individuals with Crohn's disease. Include water-rich foods and beverages to maintain hydration levels, especially during periods of increased fluid loss.

4. Cooking Methods Matter: Opt for cooking methods that enhance digestibility, such as steaming, boiling, or baking. These techniques can soften foods and make them easier to digest compared to frying or grilling.

5. Identify Trigger Foods: Keep a food diary to identify potential trigger foods that exacerbate symptoms. This can aid in tailoring your diet to individual tolerances and preferences.

6. Consider Supplements: Work with a healthcare professional to determine if nutritional supplements are necessary. Supplements can help address specific nutrient deficiencies and support overall well-being.

7. Mindful Eating: Practice mindful eating by chewing food thoroughly and savoring each bite. This aids digestion and can reduce the likelihood of gastrointestinal discomfort.

8. Plan for Flare-Ups: Have a selection of easily digestible and soothing foods on hand for times when symptoms flare. This can include items like rice, bananas, and boiled chicken.

9. Balance Macronutrients: Ensure a balanced intake of carbohydrates, proteins, and fats. This helps meet energy needs, supports overall health, and can contribute to a well-rounded diet.

10. Consult a Dietitian: Collaborate with a registered dietitian or healthcare professional specializing in gastrointestinal health. They can provide personalized guidance, taking into account individual needs and preferences.

Tailoring your approach to meal planning and preparation can significantly enhance the quality of life for individuals with Crohn's disease. Experimenting with different strategies, keeping track of what works best for you, and seeking professional guidance can empower you to create a sustainable and enjoyable dietary routine.

Guidelines for Crohn's-Friendly Eating

Adhering to Crohn's-friendly eating guidelines is crucial for managing symptoms and supporting overall well-being. Here are key recommendations to navigate a diet conducive to individuals with Crohn's disease:

1. Low-Residue Foods: Opt for easily digestible, low-residue options to minimize the amount of undigested food reaching the colon. Cooked vegetables, tender meats, and refined grains are often better tolerated.

2. Identify Trigger Foods: Keep a food journal to identify and eliminate potential trigger foods that may exacerbate symptoms. Common triggers include spicy foods, dairy, high-fiber foods, and certain fats.

3. Hydration: Stay well-hydrated to support digestion and prevent dehydration, which can be a concern during flare-ups. Choose water, herbal teas, and electrolyte-rich fluids.

4. Balanced Nutrition: Strive for a balanced intake of macronutrients—carbohydrates, proteins, and fats—to meet nutritional needs. Focus on nutrient-dense foods to support overall health.

5. Mindful Eating: Eat slowly, chew food thoroughly, and be mindful of portion sizes. This can help reduce the risk of overeating and minimize digestive discomfort.

6. Small, Frequent Meals: Opt for smaller, more frequent meals to ease the digestive process and prevent overwhelming the gastrointestinal tract. This can be particularly beneficial during periods of active disease.

7. Limit Caffeine and Alcohol: Caffeine and alcohol can irritate the digestive tract. Limiting or avoiding these substances may help manage symptoms and promote gut health.

8. Include Probiotics: Probiotics, found in certain fermented foods or supplements, can help promote a healthy balance of gut bacteria. Consult with a healthcare professional before introducing new supplements.

9. Cooking Methods: Choose gentle cooking methods such as steaming, boiling, or baking. These methods can make food more digestible compared to frying or grilling.

10. Consult with a Dietitian: Collaborate with a registered dietitian or healthcare professional

specializing in inflammatory bowel diseases. They can provide personalized advice, considering individual triggers, nutritional needs, and lifestyle factors.

Individuals with Crohn's disease may experience unique dietary requirements, and these guidelines provide a foundation for tailoring a Crohn's-friendly eating plan. Regular monitoring, openness to dietary adjustments, and professional guidance contribute to an effective and sustainable approach to managing Crohn's through nutrition.

Part II. THE RECIPES

Nutrient-packed and easy-to-digest morning option

Start your day with a nutrient-packed and easy-to-digest morning option to fuel your body and support digestive comfort. A well-balanced breakfast is essential, especially for individuals with conditions like Crohn's disease. Consider a nourishing bowl of oatmeal topped with sliced bananas, a drizzle of honey, and a sprinkle of chia seeds. Oats provide soluble fiber that is gentle on the digestive system, while bananas offer potassium, easily digestible carbohydrates, and natural sweetness. Chia seeds add omega-3 fatty acids and a delightful crunch.

Alternatively, opt for a smoothie made with easily digestible ingredients. Blend together spinach, banana, Greek yogurt, and a splash of almond milk. This smoothie provides a nutrient-packed combination of vitamins, minerals, and probiotics from the yogurt. The banana contributes natural sweetness, and spinach adds a boost of iron and fiber. The liquid nature of the smoothie makes it easy on the stomach, providing a refreshing and nutritious way to kickstart your day while promoting digestive ease.

Step By Step Process Of Making Quinoa

Creating a quinoa-based meal for individuals with Crohn's disease involves a step-by-step process that prioritizes nutrient density and ease of digestion. Here's a simple recipe for quinoa with steamed vegetables:

Ingredients:
- 1 cup quinoa
- 2 cups water or low-sodium broth
- Mixed vegetables (e.g., carrots, zucchini, bell peppers)
- Olive oil
- Salt and pepper to taste

Steps:

1. Rinse Quinoa:

Start by rinsing the quinoa under cold water to remove any residual bitterness. This step is crucial for individuals with sensitive digestive systems.

2. Cook Quinoa:

Combine the rinsed quinoa with water or low-sodium broth in a saucepan. Bring it to a boil, then reduce the heat, cover, and simmer for 15-20 minutes or until the quinoa is cooked and the liquid is absorbed.

3. Prepare Vegetables:

While the quinoa is cooking, chop the mixed vegetables into small, easily digestible pieces. Opt for well-cooked vegetables, such as steamed carrots, zucchini, and bell peppers.

4. Sauté Vegetables:

In a separate pan, lightly sauté the chopped vegetables in a small amount of olive oil. Season with a pinch of salt and pepper. This cooking method helps make the vegetables more digestible.

5. Combine Quinoa and Vegetables:

Once the quinoa is cooked, fluff it with a fork and gently mix in the sautéed vegetables. This creates a balanced dish with a variety of textures and flavors.

6. Serve Warm:

Plate the quinoa and vegetable mixture while it's still warm. For added flavor and nutritional benefits, drizzle a small amount of olive oil over the dish.

Tips:

- Portion Control: Begin with small portions and monitor how your body responds. Adjust the serving size based on individual tolerance levels.

- Customization: Tailor the recipe to individual preferences and tolerances. You can add herbs, spices, or a squeeze of lemon for extra flavor.

- Hydration: Ensure adequate hydration by drinking water or herbal teas with the meal.

This quinoa and vegetable dish offers a nutritious and easily digestible option for individuals seeking a wholesome meal that aligns with Crohn's-friendly dietary considerations.

Sep by Step Process of Making Smoothie Bowl with Greek Yogurt and Banana

Creating a nutritious and easily digestible smoothie bowl with Greek yogurt and banana for individuals with Crohn's disease involves a step-by-step process. This recipe combines the benefits of probiotic-rich yogurt, easily digestible fruits, and additional nutrients for a wholesome breakfast option.

Ingredients:
- 1 ripe banana
- 1 cup Greek yogurt (low-fat or lactose-free if needed)
- 1/2 cup berries (e.g., blueberries, raspberries)
- 1 tablespoon chia seeds
- 1 tablespoon honey (optional)
- Granola or crushed nuts for topping (optional)

Steps:

1. Prepare Ingredients:
   Gather and prepare all ingredients. Ensure the banana is ripe for natural sweetness.

2. Peel and Slice Banana:
   Peel the ripe banana and slice it into smaller pieces. This facilitates easier blending and digestion.

3. Blend Banana and Greek Yogurt:
   In a blender, combine the banana slices and Greek yogurt. Blend until smooth. Greek yogurt provides

probiotics and protein without excessive lactose, making it suitable for many individuals with Crohn's.

4. Add Berries and Chia Seeds:
   Add the berries and chia seeds to the blender. Berries offer antioxidants and natural sweetness, while chia seeds contribute omega-3 fatty acids and additional fiber.

5. Blend until Smooth:
   Blend the mixture until smooth and well combined. Adjust the consistency by adding more yogurt or a splash of water if needed.

6. Taste and Sweeten (Optional):
   Taste the smoothie and, if desired, add honey for extra sweetness. Adjust according to individual preferences and tolerances.

7. Pour into a Bowl:
   Pour the smoothie into a bowl, ensuring a smooth and even surface.

8. Top with Granola or Nuts (Optional):
   For added texture and nutritional value, top the smoothie bowl with a sprinkle of granola or crushed nuts. Choose easily digestible options based on individual preferences.

9. Serve Immediately:
   Enjoy the smoothie bowl immediately while it's fresh and chilled.

Tips:

- Temperature: If cold foods are better tolerated, consider using frozen berries or adding ice cubes to the blender.

- Hydration: Accompany the smoothie bowl with water or a soothing herbal tea to stay well-hydrated.

- Individual Adjustments: Personalize the recipe by incorporating ingredients that align with individual tolerances and preferences.

This smoothie bowl offers a delicious and nutrient-packed option for individuals seeking a gentle and satisfying breakfast.

Sep by Step Process of Making Omelette with Spinach and Feta

Creating an omelette with spinach and feta for individuals with Crohn's disease involves a gentle and nutritious approach. Here's a step-by-step process for a flavorful and easily digestible omelette:

Ingredients:
- 2 large eggs
- Handful of fresh spinach, chopped
- 2 tablespoons crumbled feta cheese
- 1 tablespoon olive oil
- Salt and pepper to taste

Steps:

1. Prepare Ingredients:
   Gather and prepare all ingredients. Ensure that the spinach is washed and chopped, and the feta cheese is crumbled.

2. Heat Olive Oil:
   Heat the olive oil in a non-stick skillet over medium heat. Use a non-stick pan to minimize the need for excess oil.

3. Sauté Spinach:
   Add the chopped spinach to the skillet. Sauté for a few minutes until the spinach wilts. Cooking the spinach ensures it's softer and easier to digest.

4. Whisk Eggs:

While the spinach is cooking, whisk the eggs in a bowl. Add a pinch of salt and pepper to taste.

5. Pour Eggs into Skillet:
   Pour the whisked eggs over the sautéed spinach in the skillet. Allow the eggs to set slightly around the edges.

6. Add Feta Cheese:
   Sprinkle the crumbled feta cheese evenly over the partially set eggs. Feta adds a burst of flavor without overwhelming the dish.

7. Fold Omelette:
   Gently lift the edges of the omelette with a spatula and fold it in half. This encases the spinach and feta within the omelette.

8. Cook Until Set:
   Continue cooking the omelette until the eggs are fully set and the feta has slightly melted. Ensure that the eggs are thoroughly cooked for easier digestion.

9. Slide onto Plate:
   Carefully slide the omelette onto a plate. The non-stick surface helps prevent sticking and tearing.

10. Serve Warm:

Serve the omelette warm. Consider pairing it with a side of well-cooked and easily digestible vegetables.

Tips:

- Low Heat: Cooking the omelette over medium heat prevents overcooking and promotes a softer texture.

- Herbs for Flavor: Consider adding fresh herbs like parsley or chives for additional flavor without increasing the load on the digestive system.

- Hydration: Accompany the omelette with a glass of water or a soothing herbal tea to aid digestion.

Sep by Step Process of Making Chia Seed Pudding with Almond Milk

Creating a gentle and nutritious chia seed pudding with almond milk for individuals with Crohn's disease involves a straightforward process. Chia seeds are a good source of omega-3 fatty acids and soluble fiber, making them a beneficial addition to a Crohn's-friendly diet. Here's a step-by-step process:

Ingredients:

- 1/4 cup chia seeds
- 1 cup unsweetened almond milk
- 1-2 tablespoons maple syrup or honey (optional, depending on sweetness preference)
- 1/2 teaspoon vanilla extract
- Fresh fruits or nuts for topping (optional)

Steps:

1. Measure Chia Seeds:
   Start by measuring 1/4 cup of chia seeds. This will be the base for the pudding.

2. Combine Chia Seeds and Almond Milk:
   In a bowl, combine the chia seeds with 1 cup of unsweetened almond milk. Stir well to ensure the chia seeds are evenly distributed.

3. Add Sweetener and Vanilla Extract:
   If desired, add 1-2 tablespoons of maple syrup or honey for sweetness. Also, include 1/2 teaspoon of vanilla extract for flavor. Adjust the sweetness according to individual preferences.

4. Stir and Let it Sit:
   Stir the mixture thoroughly to prevent clumping. Let it sit for a few minutes and then stir again to ensure the chia seeds are well dispersed.

5. Refrigerate Overnight:
   Cover the bowl and refrigerate the chia seed mixture overnight or for at least 4-6 hours. This allows the chia seeds to absorb the liquid and create a pudding-like consistency.

6. Stir Before Serving:
   Before serving, give the chia seed pudding a good stir. This step helps distribute any settled chia seeds and ensures a consistent texture.

7. Top with Fresh Fruits or Nuts (Optional):
   Optionally, top the chia seed pudding with fresh fruits like berries or sliced banana, or add a sprinkle of nuts for added texture and nutritional value.

8. Serve Chilled:
   Serve the chia seed pudding chilled. It can be enjoyed as a wholesome breakfast or a satisfying snack.

Tips:

- Texture Adjustments: If a smoother texture is preferred, blend the mixture before refrigerating. This creates a more uniform pudding consistency.

- Portion Control: Begin with a small portion to gauge individual tolerance. Adjust serving sizes based on personal preferences and digestive comfort.

- Experiment with Toppings: Customize the pudding with toppings that align with individual tolerances, such as soft fruits or finely chopped nuts.

This chia seed pudding offers a nutrient-dense and easily digestible option for individuals seeking a gentle and delicious treat.

Sep by Step Process of Making Banana Pancakes with Gluten-Free Flour

Creating banana pancakes with gluten-free flour for individuals with Crohn's disease involves a simple and stomach-friendly process. Here's a step-by-step guide to making these delicious and gentle pancakes:

Ingredients:
- 1 cup gluten-free flour mix
- 1 ripe banana, mashed
- 1 egg
- 1 cup lactose-free or non-dairy milk
- 1 tablespoon maple syrup or honey (optional)
- 1 teaspoon baking powder
- 1/2 teaspoon vanilla extract
- Pinch of salt

- Cooking oil or butter for the pan

Steps:

1. Combine Dry Ingredients:
   In a mixing bowl, combine the gluten-free flour, baking powder, and a pinch of salt. Whisk the dry ingredients together to ensure even distribution.

2. Mash the Banana:
   In a separate bowl, mash a ripe banana using a fork. The banana adds natural sweetness and moisture to the pancakes.

3. Add Wet Ingredients:
   Add the mashed banana, egg, lactose-free or non-dairy milk, vanilla extract, and optional sweetener (maple syrup or honey) to the dry ingredients. Mix until just combined. Avoid overmixing to keep the pancakes tender.

4. Let the Batter Rest:
   Allow the batter to rest for a few minutes. This helps the gluten-free flour absorb the liquid, resulting in a better texture.

5. Preheat the Pan:

Preheat a non-stick skillet or griddle over medium heat. Add a small amount of cooking oil or butter to prevent sticking.

6. Scoop and Cook:
Using a ladle or measuring cup, scoop the batter onto the preheated pan to form pancakes. Cook until bubbles form on the surface, then flip and cook the other side until golden brown.

7. Repeat the Process:
Continue scooping, flipping, and cooking until all the batter is used. Adjust the heat as needed to prevent burning.

8. Serve Warm:
Once cooked, serve the banana pancakes warm. You can top them with additional slices of banana, a drizzle of maple syrup, or a dollop of lactose-free yogurt.

Tips:

- Gluten-Free Flour Choice: Use a commercially available gluten-free flour mix or a combination of gluten-free flours like rice flour, almond flour, and tapioca flour for the pancake batter.

- Portion Control: Start with a small portion to assess individual tolerance. Adjust serving sizes based on personal preferences and digestive comfort.

- Non-Dairy Milk: Opt for lactose-free or non-dairy milk alternatives like almond milk, coconut milk, or rice milk.

These banana pancakes with gluten-free flour offer a delicious and gut-friendly breakfast option for individuals seeking a tasty yet gentle meal.

Nutrient-packed and easy-to-digest Lunch option

Crafting a nutrient-packed and easy-to-digest lunch option is vital, especially for individuals managing conditions like Crohn's disease. Consider a quinoa salad with grilled chicken, cucumber, and cherry tomatoes. Quinoa provides a high-quality protein source and is easily digestible, while the chicken adds lean protein. The cucumber and tomatoes contribute vitamins and hydration without being overly fibrous. Drizzle the salad with olive oil for healthy fats, aiding nutrient absorption. Another option is a gentle vegetable and rice soup, incorporating well-cooked carrots, zucchini, and lean protein. This warm and easily digestible meal is rich in nutrients and hydrating broth.

Sep by Step Process of Making Grilled Chicken Salad with Avocado

Creating a delicious and Crohn's-friendly Grilled Chicken Salad with Avocado involves a simple and nutritious process. Here's a step-by-step guide:

Ingredients:
- 2 boneless, skinless chicken breasts
- Mixed salad greens (e.g., spinach, arugula, or lettuce)
- 1 ripe avocado, sliced
- Cherry tomatoes, halved
- Cucumber, sliced
- Olive oil
- Lemon juice
- Salt and pepper to taste
- Fresh herbs (optional, for garnish)

Steps:

1. Preheat Grill or Grill Pan:
   Preheat your grill or grill pan over medium heat. Ensure it's well-heated before placing the chicken.

2. Season Chicken:

Season the chicken breasts with salt, pepper, and a drizzle of olive oil. This enhances flavor without adding excessive fat.

3. Grill Chicken:
Grill the chicken breasts for about 6-8 minutes per side or until fully cooked. Ensure the internal temperature reaches 165°F (74°C). Let the chicken rest for a few minutes before slicing.

4. Prepare Salad Greens:
In a large bowl, combine the mixed salad greens, halved cherry tomatoes, and sliced cucumber. These vegetables provide essential vitamins and are generally well-tolerated.

5. Slice Avocado:
Slice the ripe avocado and gently toss it with the salad greens. Avocado adds healthy fats and creaminess to the salad.

6. Slice Grilled Chicken:
Slice the grilled chicken breasts into thin strips. This ensures easy digestion and optimal distribution of protein throughout the salad.

7. Assemble Salad:

Arrange the sliced grilled chicken on top of the salad greens and avocado. Drizzle with olive oil and fresh lemon juice for a light and flavorful dressing.

8. Garnish (Optional):
   Optionally, garnish the salad with fresh herbs like parsley or cilantro for added flavor and nutritional benefits.

9. Season to Taste:
   Add additional salt and pepper to taste. Adjust the seasoning according to individual preferences and tolerances.

10. Serve Immediately:
   Serve the Grilled Chicken Salad with Avocado immediately while the chicken is warm and the flavors are fresh.

Tips:

- Hydration: Accompany the salad with water or a hydrating beverage to support digestion.

- Portion Control: Start with a moderate portion size, and adjust according to individual tolerance levels.

- Customization: Feel free to customize the salad with other tolerated vegetables or add a squeeze of lime for extra zest.

Sep by Step Process of Making Salmon and Quinoa Stuffed Bell Peppers

Creating Salmon and Quinoa Stuffed Bell Peppers, tailored for individuals with Crohn's disease, involves a careful selection of ingredients and a step-by-step process to ensure both flavor and digestibility. Here's a simple guide:

Ingredients:
- 4 large bell peppers (any color)
- 1 cup cooked quinoa
- 2 cans (6 oz each) canned salmon, drained and flaked
- 1 cup spinach, finely chopped
- 1/2 cup cherry tomatoes, diced
- 1/4 cup feta cheese, crumbled
- 2 tablespoons olive oil
- 1 teaspoon dried dill
- Salt and pepper to taste
- Lemon wedges for serving (optional)

Steps:

1. Preheat Oven:
   Preheat the oven to 375°F (190°C).

2. Prepare Bell Peppers:
   Cut the tops off the bell peppers and remove seeds
and membranes. Lightly brush the outside of the
peppers with olive oil.

3. Steam Bell Peppers:
   Place the bell peppers in a microwave-safe dish with
a small amount of water. Microwave on high for 3-4
minutes to slightly soften them. Drain any excess water.

4. Prepare Quinoa and Salmon:
   In a large bowl, combine the cooked quinoa, flaked
salmon, chopped spinach, diced cherry tomatoes,
crumbled feta cheese, olive oil, dried dill, salt, and
pepper. Mix the ingredients thoroughly.

5. Stuff Bell Peppers:
   Spoon the quinoa and salmon mixture into the
steamed bell peppers, pressing down gently to pack
the filling.

6. Bake in the Oven:

Place the stuffed bell peppers in a baking dish and bake in the preheated oven for 25-30 minutes or until the peppers are tender.

7. Serve Warm:
Once baked, remove from the oven and let them cool slightly before serving. Optionally, squeeze a bit of fresh lemon juice over the stuffed peppers for added flavor.

8. Garnish (Optional):
Garnish with additional fresh herbs, such as parsley or dill, for a burst of color and freshness.

9. Portion Control:
Serve the stuffed bell peppers in moderation to assess individual tolerance. Adjust portion sizes based on personal preferences and digestive comfort.

Tips:

- Customization: Modify the recipe by adding other tolerated vegetables or herbs according to individual preferences.

- Protein Selection: Salmon provides a rich source of omega-3 fatty acids and is generally well-tolerated. However, consider individual preferences and sensitivities when selecting protein sources.

- Hydration: Accompany the meal with water or a gentle beverage to aid digestion.

Sep by Step Process of Making Turkey and Vegetable Stir-Fry with Rice Noodles

Creating a Turkey and Vegetable Stir-Fry with Rice Noodles tailored for individuals with Crohn's disease involves selecting easily digestible ingredients and a mindful cooking process. Here's a step-by-step guide:

Ingredients:
- 8 oz rice noodles
- 1 lb ground turkey
- 2 cups mixed vegetables (e.g., bell peppers, zucchini, carrots), thinly sliced
- 2 tablespoons low-sodium soy sauce
- 1 tablespoon ginger, minced
- 2 cloves garlic, minced
- 2 tablespoons sesame oil
- Salt and pepper to taste
- Green onions (optional, for garnish)

Steps:

1. Prepare Rice Noodles:
   Cook rice noodles according to package instructions. Drain and set aside.

2. Cook Turkey:
   In a large skillet or wok, heat sesame oil over medium heat. Add ground turkey, breaking it apart with a spoon, and cook until browned.

3. Add Vegetables:
   Add thinly sliced vegetables to the skillet. Stir-fry for 3-4 minutes until they start to soften but remain crisp. Season with salt and pepper.

4. Add Ginger and Garlic:
   Stir in minced ginger and garlic, sautéing for an additional 1-2 minutes until fragrant. Be cautious with the amount of ginger if it can be irritating to the digestive system.

5. Combine Soy Sauce:
   Pour low-sodium soy sauce over the turkey and vegetable mixture. Stir well to coat evenly.

6. Add Cooked Rice Noodles:
   Add the cooked rice noodles to the skillet, tossing them with the turkey and vegetable mixture until

everything is well combined. Adjust seasoning if needed.

7. Garnish and Serve:
   Garnish the stir-fry with optional chopped green onions for freshness and additional flavor. Serve the Turkey and Vegetable Stir-Fry warm.

8. Portion Control:
   Serve in moderation to gauge individual tolerance. Adjust portion sizes based on personal preferences and digestive comfort.

Tips:

- Vegetable Variety: Include a mix of colorful vegetables for a diverse range of nutrients. Ensure they are thinly sliced for easier digestion.

- Protein Source: Turkey is a lean protein source; however, individual preferences and tolerances should guide protein choices.

- Ginger Caution: While ginger adds flavor, it may be strong for some individuals. Adjust the quantity based on personal tolerance.

- Hydration: Accompany the stir-fry with water or a gentle beverage to support digestion.

Sep by Step Process of Making Mashed Sweet Potato and Chicken Casserole

Creating a Mashed Sweet Potato and Chicken Casserole suitable for individuals with Crohn's disease involves choosing ingredients that are easily digestible and assembling them with care. Here's a step-by-step guide:

Ingredients:
- 2 large sweet potatoes, peeled and diced
- 1 lb boneless, skinless chicken breasts, cooked and shredded
- 1 cup lactose-free or non-dairy milk
- 2 tablespoons olive oil
- 1 teaspoon dried thyme
- Salt and pepper to taste
- 1/4 cup grated Parmesan cheese (optional, for topping)
- Fresh parsley (optional, for garnish)

Steps:

1. Preheat Oven:

Preheat your oven to 375°F (190°C).

2. Cook Sweet Potatoes:
   Boil or steam the peeled and diced sweet potatoes until they are tender. Drain and set aside.

3. Mash Sweet Potatoes:
   Mash the cooked sweet potatoes in a large bowl. Add lactose-free or non-dairy milk, olive oil, dried thyme, salt, and pepper. Mix until smooth. Adjust the consistency by adding more milk if needed.

4. Layer Casserole Dish:
   In a greased casserole dish, spread half of the mashed sweet potatoes as the bottom layer.

5. Add Shredded Chicken:
   Place the shredded chicken evenly over the mashed sweet potatoes layer. This provides a protein source that is gentle on the digestive system.

6. Top with Remaining Sweet Potatoes:
   Add the remaining mashed sweet potatoes as the top layer, spreading them evenly to cover the chicken.

7. Optional Parmesan Topping:
   If tolerated, sprinkle grated Parmesan cheese on top for added flavor. Adjust the quantity based on individual preferences.

8. Bake in the Oven:
   Bake the casserole in the preheated oven for 25-30 minutes or until it's heated through and the top is lightly golden.

9. Garnish and Serve:
   Garnish with fresh parsley if desired. Allow the casserole to cool slightly before serving.

10. Portion Control:
   Serve in moderation to assess individual tolerance. Adjust portion sizes based on personal preferences and digestive comfort.

Tips:

- Chicken Preparation: Ensure the chicken is cooked thoroughly before shredding to avoid any issues related to undercooked poultry.

- Milk Alternatives: Choose lactose-free or non-dairy milk alternatives based on individual tolerances. Adjust the amount to achieve the desired consistency.

- Herb Variation: Experiment with other herbs like rosemary or sage for added flavor, considering personal preferences.

- Hydration: Accompany the casserole with water or a gentle beverage to support digestion.

Sep by Step Process of Making Vegetarian Lentil Soup

Creating a Vegetarian Lentil Soup suitable for individuals with Crohn's disease involves choosing easily digestible ingredients and a gentle cooking process. Here's a step-by-step guide:

Ingredients:
- 1 cup dried green or red lentils, rinsed
- 1 large carrot, peeled and diced
- 1 celery stalk, diced
- 1 small onion, finely chopped
- 2 cloves garlic, minced
- 1 teaspoon ground cumin
- 1 teaspoon ground coriander
- 1/2 teaspoon turmeric
- 6 cups vegetable broth (low-sodium)
- 2 tablespoons olive oil
- Salt and pepper to taste
- Fresh lemon juice (optional, for serving)
- Fresh parsley (optional, for garnish)

Steps:

1. Rinse Lentils:
   Rinse the dried lentils under cold water and set them aside.

2. Sauté Vegetables:
   In a large pot, heat olive oil over medium heat. Add diced onion, carrot, and celery. Sauté until the vegetables are softened, about 5 minutes.

3. Add Garlic and Spices:
   Add minced garlic, ground cumin, ground coriander, and turmeric to the sautéed vegetables. Stir well and cook for an additional 1-2 minutes until fragrant.

4. Add Lentils and Broth:
   Pour in the rinsed lentils and vegetable broth. Bring the mixture to a boil, then reduce the heat to low, cover, and simmer for 20-25 minutes or until the lentils are tender.

5. Season to Taste:
   Season the soup with salt and pepper to taste. Adjust the seasoning based on individual preferences and tolerances.

6. Blend (Optional):

For a smoother consistency, use an immersion blender to partially blend the soup. This step is optional and can be adjusted based on personal texture preferences.

7. Serve Warm:
Ladle the Vegetarian Lentil Soup into bowls and serve it warm. Squeeze fresh lemon juice over each serving if desired.

8. Garnish (Optional):
Garnish the soup with fresh parsley for added freshness and flavor.

9. Portion Control:
Serve in moderation to gauge individual tolerance. Adjust portion sizes based on personal preferences and digestive comfort.

Tips:

- Vegetable Variations: Consider adding other well-cooked vegetables such as spinach or zucchini based on individual tolerances.

- Broth Selection: Opt for low-sodium vegetable broth to control salt intake.

- Lemon Juice: The addition of fresh lemon juice not only enhances flavor but can also aid digestion.

- Hydration: Accompany the soup with water or a soothing herbal tea to stay well-hydrated.

This Vegetarian Lentil Soup provides a gentle and nourishing option for individuals seeking a flavorful and gut-friendly meal.

Nutrient-packed and easy-to-digest Dinner option

Dinner meals for individuals managing Crohn's disease focus on easily digestible, nutrient-rich options. Grilled salmon with quinoa and steamed vegetables offers omega-3 fatty acids and protein. Alternatively, a baked chicken breast with sweet potato and green beans provides lean protein and vitamins. Vegetarian options like lentil stew with rice are rich in fiber and plant-based proteins. Portion control and customization based on individual tolerances are key, ensuring a satisfying yet gentle evening meal.

Sep by Step Process of Making Baked Cod with Lemon and Herbs

Creating Baked Cod with Lemon and Herbs for individuals with Crohn's disease involves choosing mild ingredients and a gentle cooking process. Here's a step-by-step guide:

Ingredients:
- 4 cod fillets (about 6 oz each)
- 2 tablespoons olive oil
- 2 tablespoons fresh lemon juice
- 1 teaspoon dried thyme
- 1 teaspoon dried oregano
- Salt and pepper to taste
- Lemon slices (for garnish)
- Fresh parsley (for garnish)

Steps:

1. Preheat Oven:
   Preheat your oven to 375°F (190°C).

2. Prepare Cod Fillets:
   Pat the cod fillets dry with a paper towel. Place them on a baking sheet lined with parchment paper or lightly greased.

3. Season with Herbs:
   In a small bowl, mix olive oil, fresh lemon juice, dried thyme, dried oregano, salt, and pepper. Brush the cod fillets with this herb mixture, ensuring even coverage.

4. Bake in the Oven:
   Bake the cod in the preheated oven for approximately 15-20 minutes or until the fish flakes

easily with a fork. Cooking time may vary based on the thickness of the fillets.

5. Garnish and Serve:
   Once baked, garnish the cod with fresh lemon slices and chopped parsley for a burst of flavor and freshness.

6. Portion Control:
   Serve the Baked Cod with Lemon and Herbs in moderation to assess individual tolerance. Adjust portion sizes based on personal preferences and digestive comfort.

Tips:

- Freshness of Ingredients: Use fresh cod fillets for optimal flavor and texture.

- Herb Variations: Experiment with other herbs like rosemary or dill based on personal preferences.

- Lemon Garnish: Lemon adds a refreshing element and can aid digestion. Adjust the quantity based on individual tolerance.

- Hydration: Accompany the cod with water or a gentle beverage to support digestion.

This Baked Cod with Lemon and Herbs offers a light and flavorful option for individuals seeking a delicious and gut-friendly dinner.

Sep by Step Process of Making Zucchini Noodles with Tomato Sauce and Grilled Shrimp

Creating Zucchini Noodles with Tomato Sauce and Grilled Shrimp for individuals with Crohn's disease involves incorporating gentle ingredients and careful preparation. Here's a step-by-step guide:

Ingredients:
- 4 medium-sized zucchinis, spiralized into noodles
- 1 lb large shrimp, peeled and deveined
- 2 cups tomato sauce (low-acid, low-sugar)
- 2 tablespoons olive oil
- 2 cloves garlic, minced
- 1 teaspoon dried basil
- 1 teaspoon dried oregano
- Salt and pepper to taste
- Fresh basil leaves (for garnish)

Steps:

1. Prepare Zucchini Noodles:

Spiralize the zucchinis into noodle shapes. Set aside.

2. Grill Shrimp:
   Season the peeled and deveined shrimp with olive oil, minced garlic, dried basil, dried oregano, salt, and pepper. Grill the shrimp until they are cooked through and have a light char, usually 2-3 minutes per side.

3. Make Tomato Sauce:
   In a separate pan, heat the tomato sauce over medium heat. Add additional herbs or spices if desired, keeping in mind individual tolerances.

4. Sauté Zucchini Noodles:
   In a large skillet, heat a small amount of olive oil. Sauté the zucchini noodles for 2-3 minutes until they are just tender but still have a slight crunch.

5. Combine Ingredients:
   Add the grilled shrimp to the skillet with zucchini noodles. Pour the tomato sauce over the mixture and gently toss until everything is well coated and heated through.

6. Season to Taste:
   Adjust the seasoning with salt and pepper to taste. Be mindful of individual preferences and sensitivities.

7. Serve Warm:

Dish out the Zucchini Noodles with Tomato Sauce and Grilled Shrimp onto plates. Garnish with fresh basil leaves for added flavor and presentation.

8. Portion Control:
   Serve in moderation to assess individual tolerance. Adjust portion sizes based on personal preferences and digestive comfort.

Tips:

- Zucchini Texture: Be cautious not to overcook the zucchini noodles to maintain a desirable texture.

- Low-Acid Tomato Sauce: Choose a tomato sauce that is low in acidity and sugar to minimize potential digestive discomfort.

- Alternative Protein: For those who prefer alternatives to shrimp, consider grilled chicken or tofu as protein options.

- Hydration: Accompany the dish with water or a gentle beverage to support digestion.

This Zucchini Noodles with Tomato Sauce and Grilled Shrimp recipe offers a flavorful and easily digestible option for individuals seeking a satisfying and gut-friendly meal.

Sep by Step Process of Making Crockpot Chicken and Vegetable Stew

Creating a Crockpot Chicken and Vegetable Stew for individuals with Crohn's disease involves selecting easily digestible ingredients and utilizing a gentle cooking process. Here's a step-by-step guide:

Ingredients:
- 1.5 lbs boneless, skinless chicken thighs, cut into bite-sized pieces
- 4 cups low-sodium chicken broth
- 4 carrots, peeled and sliced
- 2 parsnips, peeled and sliced
- 2 potatoes, peeled and diced
- 1 cup green beans, trimmed and chopped
- 1 cup celery, sliced
- 1 onion, finely chopped
- 2 cloves garlic, minced
- 1 teaspoon dried thyme
- 1 teaspoon dried rosemary
- Salt and pepper to taste
- 2 tablespoons olive oil
- Fresh parsley (optional, for garnish)

Steps:

1. Sauté Chicken:
  In a skillet, heat olive oil over medium-high heat. Brown the chicken pieces on all sides until they develop a golden color. Transfer the chicken to the slow cooker.

2. Prepare Vegetables:
  Add carrots, parsnips, potatoes, green beans, celery, onion, and garlic to the slow cooker with the browned chicken.

3. Season with Herbs:
  Sprinkle dried thyme, dried rosemary, salt, and pepper over the chicken and vegetables.

4. Pour Chicken Broth:
  Pour low-sodium chicken broth over the chicken and vegetables in the slow cooker. Ensure the ingredients are well-submerged.

5. Cook in the Crockpot:
  Set the slow cooker to low heat and cook for 6-8 hours or until the chicken and vegetables are tender. Alternatively, cook on high heat for 3-4 hours.

6. Check Seasoning:

Taste the stew and adjust the seasoning with additional salt and pepper if needed.

7. Serve Warm:
   Ladle the Crockpot Chicken and Vegetable Stew into bowls. Garnish with fresh parsley if desired.

8. Portion Control:
   Serve in moderation to assess individual tolerance. Adjust portion sizes based on personal preferences and digestive comfort.

Tips:

- Chicken Thighs: Opt for boneless, skinless chicken thighs for tenderness and flavor.

- Vegetable Selection: Include easily digestible vegetables like carrots, parsnips, and green beans. Customize based on individual tolerances.

- Low-Sodium Broth: Choose low-sodium chicken broth to control salt intake.

- Herb Variations: Experiment with other herbs like sage or parsley based on personal preferences.

- Hydration: Accompany the stew with water or a gentle beverage to support digestion.

This Crockpot Chicken and Vegetable Stew provides a comforting and nutrient-rich option for individuals seeking a flavorful and gut-friendly meal.

Sep by Step Process of Making Quinoa and Roasted Vegetable Bowl

Creating a Quinoa and Roasted Vegetable Bowl for individuals with Crohn's disease involves selecting easily digestible ingredients and utilizing a careful cooking process. Here's a step-by-step guide:

Ingredients:
- 1 cup quinoa, rinsed
- 2 cups mixed vegetables (zucchini, bell peppers, cherry tomatoes, etc.), diced
- 2 tablespoons olive oil
- 1 teaspoon dried oregano
- 1 teaspoon dried thyme
- Salt and pepper to taste
- 1/4 cup feta cheese, crumbled (optional, for topping)
- Fresh parsley or basil (optional, for garnish)

Steps:

1. Preheat Oven:
   Preheat your oven to 400°F (200°C).

2. Prepare Quinoa:
   Rinse the quinoa under cold water. Cook the quinoa according to package instructions. Set aside.

3. Dice Vegetables:
   Dice the mixed vegetables into bite-sized pieces. Aim for uniform sizes for even roasting.

4. Toss Vegetables:
   In a bowl, toss the diced vegetables with olive oil, dried oregano, dried thyme, salt, and pepper until evenly coated.

5. Roast Vegetables:
   Spread the seasoned vegetables on a baking sheet lined with parchment paper. Roast in the preheated oven for 20-25 minutes or until they are tender and slightly caramelized.

6. Fluff Quinoa:
   Fluff the cooked quinoa with a fork to separate the grains.

7. Assemble Bowl:
   In serving bowls, layer the cooked quinoa with the roasted vegetables.

8. Top with Feta (Optional):
   Sprinkle crumbled feta cheese over the quinoa and vegetables for added flavor. Adjust the quantity based on individual preferences.

9. Garnish (Optional):
   Garnish the bowl with fresh parsley or basil for a burst of freshness.

10. Portion Control:
   Serve the Quinoa and Roasted Vegetable Bowl in moderation to assess individual tolerance. Adjust portion sizes based on personal preferences and digestive comfort.

Tips:

- Vegetable Selection: Choose easily digestible vegetables and consider personal tolerances when selecting varieties.

- Quinoa Cooking: Cook quinoa with a 2:1 ratio of water to quinoa for optimal texture.

- Feta Cheese: If tolerated, feta cheese adds a creamy and tangy element to the bowl.

- Herb Variations: Experiment with other herbs like rosemary or cumin based on personal preferences.

- Hydration: Accompany the bowl with water or a gentle beverage to support digestion.

This Quinoa and Roasted Vegetable Bowl offers a flavorful and easily digestible option for individuals seeking a nutritious and gut-friendly meal.

Sep by Step Process of Making Baked Eggplant Parmesan with Gluten-Free Breadcrumbs

Creating Baked Eggplant Parmesan with Gluten-Free Breadcrumbs for individuals with Crohn's disease involves choosing easily digestible ingredients and a gentle cooking process. Here's a step-by-step guide:

Ingredients:
- 1 large eggplant, thinly sliced
- 1 cup gluten-free breadcrumbs
- 1/2 cup grated Parmesan cheese
- 2 eggs, beaten
- 2 cups marinara sauce (low-acid, low-sugar)
- 1 cup shredded mozzarella cheese
- 2 tablespoons olive oil

- Fresh basil (optional, for garnish)
- Salt and pepper to taste

Steps:

1. Preheat Oven:
   Preheat your oven to 400°F (200°C).

2. Prepare Eggplant:
   Thinly slice the eggplant into rounds. Sprinkle the slices with salt and let them sit for 15-20 minutes to release excess moisture. Pat them dry with a paper towel.

3. Set Up Breading Station:
   In separate bowls, place gluten-free breadcrumbs and beaten eggs. Dip each eggplant slice into the beaten eggs, then coat with gluten-free breadcrumbs.

4. Bake Eggplant:
   Place the breaded eggplant slices on a baking sheet lined with parchment paper. Bake in the preheated oven for 15-20 minutes or until they are golden brown and crispy.

5. Assemble Parmesan Layers:
   In a baking dish, layer the baked eggplant slices with marinara sauce, grated Parmesan cheese, and shredded mozzarella cheese.

6. Repeat Layers:
   Repeat the layers until all the ingredients are used, finishing with a layer of mozzarella cheese on top.

7. Drizzle with Olive Oil:
   Drizzle the top with olive oil to aid in browning during baking.

8. Bake in the Oven:
   Bake the Baked Eggplant Parmesan in the preheated oven for 25-30 minutes or until the cheese is melted and bubbly.

9. Garnish (Optional):
   Garnish with fresh basil leaves for added flavor and presentation.

10. Portion Control:
   Serve in moderation to assess individual tolerance. Adjust portion sizes based on personal preferences and digestive comfort.

Tips:

- Eggplant Slicing: Uniform slicing ensures even cooking. Choose smaller eggplants for tender slices.

- Gluten-Free Breadcrumbs: Opt for gluten-free breadcrumbs to accommodate dietary restrictions.

- Low-Acid Marinara Sauce: Choose a low-acid and low-sugar marinara sauce to minimize potential digestive discomfort.

- Cheese Amount: Adjust the quantity of cheese based on individual tolerances.

- Hydration: Accompany the dish with water or a gentle beverage to support digestion.

This Baked Eggplant Parmesan with Gluten-Free Breadcrumbs offers a flavorful and easily digestible option for individuals seeking a comforting and gut-friendly meal.

Nutrient-packed and easy-to-digest Snack ideas

Snack ideas for individuals managing Crohn's disease focus on simplicity and digestibility. Consider options like plain rice cakes with almond butter for a balanced snack. Greek yogurt with ripe banana slices provides probiotics and potassium. Steamed and cooled sweet potato wedges offer a nutrient-dense, easy-to-digest alternative. Smooth nut butters or hummus paired with gluten-free crackers are convenient and satisfying. Portion control is key, ensuring snacks are gentle on the digestive system.

Sep by Step Process of Making Greek Yogurt with Honey and Almonds

Creating Greek Yogurt with Honey and Almonds for individuals with Crohn's disease involves selecting gentle ingredients and a mindful preparation process. Here's a step-by-step guide:

Ingredients:
- 1 cup plain Greek yogurt (lactose-free, if needed)
- 1 tablespoon honey (or to taste)
- 2 tablespoons almonds, sliced or chopped
- Fresh berries (optional, for garnish)

Steps:

1. Select Yogurt:
   Choose a plain Greek yogurt that is suitable for individuals with lactose intolerance, ensuring it contains live and active cultures for added probiotic benefits.

2. Prepare Almonds:
   Slice or chop almonds into smaller pieces for easy digestion. Toasting them lightly can enhance flavor but is optional.

3. Assemble Yogurt Bowl:
   Spoon the Greek yogurt into a bowl. Drizzle honey over the yogurt, adjusting the quantity based on sweetness preferences.

4. Add Almonds:
   Sprinkle the sliced or chopped almonds over the yogurt and honey.

5. Garnish (Optional):

Optionally, garnish with fresh berries for added color and a burst of natural sweetness.

6. Serve Immediately:
Enjoy the Greek Yogurt with Honey and Almonds immediately for optimal texture and flavor.

7. Portion Control:
Serve in moderation to assess individual tolerance. Adjust portion sizes based on personal preferences and digestive comfort.

Tips:

- Honey Quantity: Customize the amount of honey based on individual sweetness preferences and tolerances.

- Nut Variety: Experiment with other easily digestible nuts, such as walnuts or pecans, based on personal preferences.

- Fresh Berries: Berries can provide antioxidants and additional natural sweetness. Choose low-acid varieties if necessary.

- Hydration: Accompany the yogurt with water or a gentle beverage to support digestion.

This Greek Yogurt with Honey and Almonds offers a delicious and easily digestible snack or breakfast option for individuals seeking a nourishing and gut-friendly choice.

Sep by Step Process of Making Rice Cakes with Peanut Butter and Sliced Banana

Creating Rice Cakes with Peanut Butter and Sliced Banana for individuals with Crohn's disease involves choosing gentle ingredients and a straightforward assembly. Here's a step-by-step guide:

Ingredients:
- Rice cakes (gluten-free, if needed)
- Natural peanut butter (unsweetened)
- Ripe banana, thinly sliced
- Honey (optional, for drizzling)
- Cinnamon (optional, for sprinkling)

Steps:

1. Select Rice Cakes:
   Choose plain rice cakes, ensuring they are gluten-free if necessary, for a gentle base.

2. Spread Peanut Butter:
   Spread a layer of natural peanut butter on each rice cake. Opt for an unsweetened variety to minimize added sugars.

3. Slice Banana:
   Thinly slice a ripe banana into rounds.

4. Arrange Banana Slices:
   Arrange banana slices on top of the peanut butter-covered rice cakes evenly.

5. Optional Drizzle:
   Drizzle a small amount of honey over the banana slices for added sweetness. Adjust the quantity based on personal preferences.

6. Optional Cinnamon Sprinkle:
   Optionally, sprinkle a dash of cinnamon over the assembled rice cakes for additional flavor.

7. Serve Immediately:
   Enjoy the Rice Cakes with Peanut Butter and Sliced Banana immediately for optimal texture and freshness.

8. Portion Control:
   Serve in moderation to assess individual tolerance. Adjust portion sizes based on personal preferences and digestive comfort.

Tips:

- Peanut Butter Choice: Opt for natural peanut butter without added sugars or hydrogenated oils for a healthier option.

- Banana Ripeness: Use ripe bananas for natural sweetness and easier digestion.

- Honey Usage: If tolerated, honey can add sweetness. Adjust the quantity based on individual preferences and tolerances.

- Cinnamon Addition: Cinnamon not only enhances flavor but may also have anti-inflammatory properties. Use in moderation.

- Hydration: Accompany the rice cakes with water or a gentle beverage to support digestion.

This Rice Cakes with Peanut Butter and Sliced Banana recipe offers a quick, satisfying, and gut-friendly snack for individuals seeking a nutritious and easily digestible option.

Sep by Step Process of Making Homemade Trail Mix with Seeds and Dried Fruits

Creating a Homemade Trail Mix with Seeds and Dried Fruits for individuals with Crohn's disease involves selecting easily digestible ingredients and combining them with care. Here's a step-by-step guide:

Ingredients:
- 1 cup pumpkin seeds (pepitas)
- 1 cup sunflower seeds
- 1 cup almonds, chopped
- 1 cup dried cranberries
- 1 cup dried apricots, chopped
- 1/2 cup unsweetened coconut flakes
- 1/2 cup dark chocolate chips (optional)
- 1 teaspoon cinnamon (optional)
- 1/2 teaspoon sea salt (optional)

Steps:

1. Preheat Oven (Optional):
   If desired, preheat your oven to 325°F (163°C) for toasting the seeds. Toasting adds flavor but is optional.

2. Toast Seeds (Optional):

In a dry skillet over medium heat, toast pumpkin seeds and sunflower seeds until they become fragrant, stirring frequently. Remove from heat and let them cool.

3. Combine Ingredients:
   In a large mixing bowl, combine the toasted seeds, chopped almonds, dried cranberries, chopped dried apricots, unsweetened coconut flakes, and dark chocolate chips if using.

4. Optional Seasoning:
   Add cinnamon and sea salt if desired. Adjust quantities based on personal preferences.

5. Mix Thoroughly:
   Mix all the ingredients thoroughly to ensure an even distribution of flavors.

6. Store in an Airtight Container:
   Transfer the Homemade Trail Mix to an airtight container to preserve freshness. Shake or stir occasionally to prevent ingredients from settling.

7. Portion Control:
   Portion the trail mix into smaller snack-sized containers for convenient and controlled servings.

8. Serve as Needed:

Enjoy the trail mix as a snack, on its own, or as a topping for yogurt or oatmeal.

Tips:

- Seed and Nut Choices: Choose easily digestible seeds and nuts, such as pumpkin seeds, sunflower seeds, and chopped almonds.

- Dried Fruit Selection: Opt for easily digestible dried fruits like cranberries and chopped apricots. Avoid those with added sugars or sulfites.

- Chocolate Consideration: If using chocolate chips, choose dark chocolate for potential antioxidant benefits.

- Cinnamon and Salt: These are optional additions for flavor enhancement. Use in moderation.

- Hydration: Accompany the trail mix with water or a gentle beverage to support digestion.

This Homemade Trail Mix with Seeds and Dried Fruits offers a convenient and nutrient-rich snack for individuals seeking a flavorful and easily digestible option.

Sep by Step Process of Making Baked Apple Chips

Creating Baked Apple Chips for individuals with Crohn's disease involves choosing easily digestible ingredients and using a simple preparation process. Here's a step-by-step guide:

Ingredients:
- 4 apples (any variety, preferably with thin skin)
- 1 teaspoon ground cinnamon
- 1 tablespoon sugar or sweetener of choice (optional)
- Cooking spray or a light coating of olive oil

Steps:

1. Preheat Oven:
   Preheat your oven to 200°F (93°C). This low temperature helps dehydrate the apples slowly, preserving their nutritional value.

2. Wash and Slice Apples:
   Wash the apples thoroughly. Core the apples and slice them into thin, even rounds, about 1/8 inch thick. Removing the peel is optional, depending on individual preferences and tolerances.

3. Coat with Cinnamon and Sweetener (Optional):
   In a bowl, toss the apple slices with ground cinnamon. Add sugar or a sweetener of choice if desired. Adjust sweetness based on personal preferences.

4. Prepare Baking Sheets:
   Line baking sheets with parchment paper or lightly coat them with cooking spray.

5. Arrange Apple Slices:
   Arrange the apple slices in a single layer on the prepared baking sheets. Ensure they are not touching to allow even dehydration.

6. Bake in the Oven:
   Bake the apple slices in the preheated oven for 2-3 hours, flipping them halfway through. Baking time may vary based on the thickness of the slices.

7. Check for Crispiness:
   Check for crispiness by testing a cooled apple slice. They should be firm and crunchy but not overly dry.

8. Cool Completely:
   Allow the Baked Apple Chips to cool completely on a wire rack before storing to maintain their crisp texture.

9. Store in an Airtight Container:

Once cooled, store the apple chips in an airtight container to preserve their crunchiness.

10. Serve as Needed:
   Enjoy the Baked Apple Chips as a snack or use them as a topping for yogurt, oatmeal, or desserts.

Tips:

- Apple Variety: Choose apple varieties with thin skin for a more delicate chip. Experiment with different varieties for diverse flavors.

- Thin and Even Slicing: Aim for thin and even slices to ensure uniform dehydration.

- Peeling Option: Peeling is optional; leaving the peel on adds extra fiber and nutrients.

- Sweetener Consideration: Use sweeteners sparingly or omit entirely for a naturally sweet flavor.

- Cinnamon Amount: Adjust the amount of cinnamon based on personal preferences.

- Hydration: Enjoy the apple chips with water or a gentle beverage to support digestion.

These Baked Apple Chips provide a delightful and gut-friendly snack for individuals seeking a crunchy and nutritious option.

Sep by Step Process of Making Vegetable Sticks with Hummus

Creating Vegetable Sticks with Hummus for individuals with Crohn's disease involves choosing easily digestible vegetables and using a gentle hummus recipe. Here's a step-by-step guide:

Ingredients:

Vegetable Sticks:
- 2 large carrots, peeled and cut into sticks
- 2 bell peppers (assorted colors), sliced into strips
- 2 cucumbers, cut into sticks
- 1 zucchini, sliced into sticks
- 1 cup cherry tomatoes, halved
- Other vegetables of choice

Hummus:
- 1 can (15 oz) chickpeas, drained and rinsed
- 2 cloves garlic, minced
- 3 tablespoons tahini

- 3 tablespoons lemon juice
- 2 tablespoons olive oil
- 1/2 teaspoon ground cumin
- Salt and pepper to taste
- Water (as needed for consistency)

Steps:

1. Prepare Vegetables:
   Wash, peel (if needed), and cut the vegetables into stick shapes. Ensure they are easily manageable for dipping.

2. Make Hummus:
   In a food processor, combine chickpeas, minced garlic, tahini, lemon juice, olive oil, ground cumin, salt, and pepper. Blend until smooth. Add water as needed for a smoother consistency.

3. Arrange Vegetable Sticks:
   Arrange the vegetable sticks on a serving platter or individual plates.

4. Serve with Hummus:
   Place the freshly made hummus in a bowl or several small bowls for individual servings.

5. Garnish (Optional):

Optionally, garnish the hummus with a drizzle of olive oil, a sprinkle of cumin, or a few whole chickpeas for visual appeal.

6. Portion Control:
Serve the Vegetable Sticks with Hummus in moderation to assess individual tolerance. Adjust portion sizes based on personal preferences and digestive comfort.

7. Enjoy as a Snack or Appetizer:
Enjoy the Vegetable Sticks with Hummus as a nutritious snack or appetizer.

Tips:

- Vegetable Selection: Choose easily digestible vegetables, and consider personal tolerances when selecting varieties.

- Hummus Texture: Adjust the water content in the hummus to achieve the desired thickness.

- Garnish Options: Experiment with garnishes like chopped fresh herbs, paprika, or a squeeze of additional lemon juice.

- Hydration: Accompany the snack with water or a gentle beverage to support digestion.

This Vegetable Sticks with Hummus recipe provides a tasty and gut-friendly option for individuals seeking a light and nutritious snack.

Nutrient-packed and easy-to-digest Dessert indulgences

Dessert indulgences for individuals with Crohn's disease can be both satisfying and gentle on the digestive system. Opt for treats like a ripe banana with a drizzle of honey, providing natural sweetness and potassium. Chilled fruit sorbets or lactose-free frozen yogurt offer a refreshing alternative. Dark chocolate, in moderation, can satisfy sweet cravings with potential antioxidant benefits. Desserts can be tailored to individual tolerances, emphasizing simple ingredients and mindful portion control.

Sep by Step Process of Making Banana and Coconut Milk Ice Cream

Creating Banana and Coconut Milk Ice Cream for individuals with Crohn's disease involves selecting gentle ingredients and utilizing a simple preparation process. Here's a step-by-step guide:

Ingredients:

- 4 ripe bananas, peeled and sliced
- 1 can (13.5 oz) coconut milk (full-fat or lite)
- 1 teaspoon vanilla extract (optional)
- 2 tablespoons honey or maple syrup (optional, for added sweetness)

Steps:

1. Freeze Banana Slices:
   Peel and slice ripe bananas. Place the banana slices in a single layer on a tray or plate and freeze until solid, ideally overnight.

2. Blend Frozen Bananas:
   In a blender or food processor, combine the frozen banana slices, coconut milk, vanilla extract (if using), and honey or maple syrup (if adding sweetness). Blend until smooth and creamy.

3. Adjust Consistency:
   If the mixture is too thick, you can add a bit more coconut milk to achieve the desired ice cream consistency.

4. Serve Immediately or Freeze:

Serve the Banana and Coconut Milk Ice Cream immediately for a soft-serve texture, or transfer the mixture to a container and freeze for a couple of hours for a firmer consistency.

5. Portion Control:
   Serve in moderation to assess individual tolerance. Adjust portion sizes based on personal preferences and digestive comfort.

6. Garnish (Optional):
   Optionally, garnish the ice cream with shredded coconut, sliced bananas, or a drizzle of honey before serving.

7. Enjoy Responsibly:
   Enjoy the Banana and Coconut Milk Ice Cream as a delicious and gut-friendly dessert.

Tips:

- Banana Ripeness: Choose ripe bananas for natural sweetness. The riper they are, the sweeter the ice cream.

- Coconut Milk Options: Opt for full-fat or lite coconut milk based on individual preferences and tolerances.

- Sweetener Choice: Adjust the sweetness by adding honey, maple syrup, or other sweeteners, keeping in mind individual preferences and digestive considerations.

- Variations: Experiment with flavor variations by adding a pinch of cinnamon, a splash of lime juice, or a handful of frozen berries to the blend.

- Hydration: Enjoy the ice cream with water or a gentle beverage to support digestion.

This Banana and Coconut Milk Ice Cream offers a delightful and easily digestible dessert option for those seeking a sweet treat while considering their digestive health.

Sep by Step Process of Making Chocolate Avocado Mousse

Creating Chocolate Avocado Mousse for individuals with Crohn's disease involves selecting gentle ingredients and using a simple preparation process. Here's a step-by-step guide:

Ingredients:

- 2 ripe avocados, peeled and pitted
- 1/2 cup unsweetened cocoa powder
- 1/2 cup maple syrup or honey
- 1/4 cup coconut milk or lactose-free milk
- 1 teaspoon vanilla extract
- Pinch of salt
- Optional toppings: berries, shredded coconut, or chopped nuts

Steps:

1. Prepare Avocados:
   Peel and pit the ripe avocados, ensuring only the creamy green flesh is used.

2. Blend Ingredients:
   In a blender or food processor, combine the avocado flesh, cocoa powder, maple syrup or honey, coconut milk or lactose-free milk, vanilla extract, and a pinch of salt.

3. Blend Until Smooth:
   Blend the ingredients until the mixture becomes smooth and creamy. Stop and scrape down the sides of the blender or processor if needed.

4. Adjust Sweetness:

Taste the mousse and adjust the sweetness by adding more maple syrup or honey if desired.

5. Chill (Optional):

For a firmer texture, you can chill the Chocolate Avocado Mousse in the refrigerator for an hour or more before serving.

6. Portion Control:

Serve in moderation to assess individual tolerance. Adjust portion sizes based on personal preferences and digestive comfort.

7. Garnish (Optional):

Optionally, garnish the mousse with fresh berries, shredded coconut, or chopped nuts before serving.

8. Enjoy Responsibly:

Enjoy the Chocolate Avocado Mousse as a rich and satisfying dessert.

Tips:

- Avocado Ripeness: Ensure the avocados are ripe for a smooth texture and optimal flavor.

- Cocoa Powder Selection: Choose unsweetened cocoa powder to control the sweetness level.

- Sweetener Choice: Adjust the sweetness by using maple syrup or honey, considering individual preferences and digestive considerations.

- Milk Alternative: Opt for coconut milk or lactose-free milk for a dairy-free option.

- Variations: Experiment with flavor variations by adding a pinch of cinnamon, a dash of coffee extract, or a hint of orange zest.

- Hydration: Enjoy the mousse with water or a gentle beverage to support digestion.

This Chocolate Avocado Mousse offers a decadent and easily digestible dessert option for those with digestive health in mind.

Sep by Step Process of Making Almond Flour Blueberry Muffins

Creating Almond Flour Blueberry Muffins for individuals with Crohn's disease involves using easily digestible ingredients and a careful baking process. Here's a step-by-step guide:

Ingredients:

- 2 cups almond flour
- 1/4 cup coconut flour
- 1/2 teaspoon baking soda
- 1/4 teaspoon salt
- 3 large eggs
- 1/4 cup coconut oil, melted
- 1/4 cup honey or maple syrup
- 1 teaspoon vanilla extract
- 1 cup fresh or frozen blueberries

Steps:

1. Preheat Oven:
   Preheat your oven to 350°F (175°C). Line a muffin tin with paper liners.

2. Mix Dry Ingredients:
   In a bowl, combine almond flour, coconut flour, baking soda, and salt. Mix well to ensure even distribution.

3. Whisk Wet Ingredients:
   In another bowl, whisk together the eggs, melted coconut oil, honey or maple syrup, and vanilla extract until well combined.

4. Combine Wet and Dry Mixtures:

Pour the wet ingredients into the bowl with the dry ingredients. Mix until just combined, avoiding overmixing.

5. Fold in Blueberries:
   Gently fold in the blueberries into the batter, ensuring even distribution.

6. Fill Muffin Cups:
   Spoon the batter into the prepared muffin cups, filling each about two-thirds full.

7. Bake in the Oven:
   Bake in the preheated oven for 18-22 minutes or until a toothpick inserted into the center of a muffin comes out clean.

8. Cool Muffins:
   Allow the Almond Flour Blueberry Muffins to cool in the muffin tin for 5 minutes, then transfer them to a wire rack to cool completely.

9. Portion Control:
   Serve the muffins in moderation to assess individual tolerance. Adjust portion sizes based on personal preferences and digestive comfort.

10. Enjoy Responsibly:

Enjoy the Almond Flour Blueberry Muffins as a tasty and gut-friendly treat.

Tips:

- Almond Flour Quality: Choose high-quality almond flour for a finer texture.

- Blueberry Selection: Use fresh or frozen blueberries, and consider individual tolerances when selecting varieties.

- Oil Choice: Coconut oil adds a subtle flavor, but you can use another mild oil if preferred.

- Sweetener Amount: Adjust the amount of honey or maple syrup based on personal sweetness preferences.

- Storage: Store muffins in an airtight container in the refrigerator for freshness.

- Hydration: Enjoy the muffins with water or a gentle beverage to support digestion.

These Almond Flour Blueberry Muffins offer a delicious and easily digestible baked good for those mindful of their digestive health.

Sep by Step Process of Making Baked Pears with Cinnamon and Walnuts

Creating Baked Pears with Cinnamon and Walnuts for individuals with Crohn's disease involves selecting gentle ingredients and a simple baking process. Here's a step-by-step guide:

Ingredients:

- 4 ripe but firm pears, halved and cored
- 1 tablespoon lemon juice
- 1 teaspoon ground cinnamon
- 1/4 cup chopped walnuts
- 2 tablespoons honey or maple syrup (optional)
- 1 tablespoon coconut oil, melted (or alternative mild oil)
- Pinch of salt

Steps:

1. Preheat Oven:
   Preheat your oven to 375°F (190°C).

2. Prepare Pears:

Halve and core the ripe but firm pears. Brush the cut sides with lemon juice to prevent browning.

3. Arrange Pears in Baking Dish:
   Place the pear halves, cut side up, in a baking dish.

4. Combine Cinnamon and Walnuts:
   In a small bowl, mix together the ground cinnamon and chopped walnuts.

5. Fill Pears:
   Sprinkle the cinnamon and walnut mixture evenly over the cut sides of the pears.

6. Optional Sweetener:
   Drizzle honey or maple syrup over the pears for added sweetness, if desired.

7. Drizzle with Coconut Oil:
   Drizzle melted coconut oil (or an alternative mild oil) over the pears. This adds moisture and enhances flavor.

8. Bake in the Oven:
   Bake the pears in the preheated oven for 25-30 minutes or until the pears are tender and the tops are lightly browned.

9. Check for Doneness:

Test the pears with a fork to ensure they are tender but not mushy.

10. Serve Warm:
   Serve the Baked Pears with Cinnamon and Walnuts warm, optionally with a dollop of yogurt or a sprinkle of additional cinnamon.

Tips:

- Pear Selection: Choose ripe but firm pears to ensure they hold their shape during baking.

- Nut Variety: Experiment with other easily digestible nuts, such as almonds or pecans, based on personal preferences.

- Sweetener Amount: Adjust the amount of honey or maple syrup based on personal sweetness preferences.

- Oil Choice: Coconut oil adds a subtle flavor, but you can use another mild oil if preferred.

- Serve with Yogurt: Adding a dollop of yogurt on top can enhance the creaminess and add a touch of tang.

- Hydration: Enjoy the baked pears with water or a gentle beverage to support digestion.

These Baked Pears with Cinnamon and Walnuts offer a delightful and easily digestible dessert option for those mindful of their digestive health.

Sep by Step Process of Making Chia Seed and Berry Parfait

Creating a Chia Seed and Berry Parfait for individuals with Crohn's disease involves selecting gentle ingredients and a simple assembly process. Here's a step-by-step guide:

Ingredients:

- 3 tablespoons chia seeds
- 1 cup lactose-free yogurt or non-dairy alternative
- 1 tablespoon honey or maple syrup (optional)
- 1 teaspoon vanilla extract (optional)
- Mixed berries (e.g., strawberries, blueberries, raspberries)
- 1/4 cup granola (gluten-free if needed)
- Fresh mint leaves for garnish (optional)

Steps:

1. Prepare Chia Pudding:

In a bowl, mix chia seeds with lactose-free yogurt or a non-dairy alternative. Add honey or maple syrup and vanilla extract if desired. Stir well and let it sit in the refrigerator for at least 2 hours or overnight to thicken.

2. Assemble Parfait:
Take the chia pudding out of the refrigerator. In serving glasses or bowls, layer the chia pudding with mixed berries.

3. Add Granola:
Sprinkle a layer of granola on top of the berries. Granola adds crunch and additional texture.

4. Repeat Layers:
Repeat the layering process until the glass or bowl is filled, finishing with a layer of berries and a sprinkle of granola on top.

5. Garnish (Optional):
Optionally, garnish the Chia Seed and Berry Parfait with fresh mint leaves for a burst of color and added freshness.

6. Serve Immediately:
Serve the parfait immediately to enjoy the contrasting textures and flavors.

7. Portion Control:

Serve in moderation to assess individual tolerance. Adjust portion sizes based on personal preferences and digestive comfort.

8. Enjoy Responsibly:
   Enjoy the Chia Seed and Berry Parfait as a nutritious and gut-friendly dessert or breakfast option.

Tips:

- Chia Seed Quality: Choose high-quality chia seeds for better texture in the pudding.

- Yogurt or Alternative: Opt for lactose-free yogurt or a non-dairy alternative based on individual preferences and tolerances.

- Sweetener Consideration: Adjust the sweetness by adding honey or maple syrup, keeping in mind individual sweetness preferences.

- Berry Selection: Use a variety of berries for added color, flavor, and nutritional diversity.

- Granola Choice: Choose a gluten-free granola if needed and select a low-sugar option.

- Hydration: Enjoy the parfait with water or a gentle beverage to support digestion.

This Chia Seed and Berry Parfait provides a delicious and easily digestible option for those mindful of their digestive health.

Cooking Techniques and Tips

For individuals navigating Crohn's disease, adopting specific cooking techniques and tips can significantly enhance their culinary experience while promoting digestive comfort. Here's a guide tailored to accommodate the unique needs of those managing Crohn's:

Gentle Cooking Techniques:

1. Steaming and Poaching: Opt for gentle cooking methods like steaming or poaching to retain the nutritional value of ingredients while ensuring they are easy on the digestive system.

2. Blending and Pureeing: Transforming foods into smooth textures through blending or pureeing can make them more digestible, offering a pleasant alternative for those with sensitive digestive systems.

3. Grilling and Roasting: Grilling and roasting allow for the development of rich flavors without excessive use of oils or fats, providing a savory appeal while being mindful of potential trigger ingredients.

Digestive-Friendly Tips:

1. Fiber Management: Tailor fiber intake by choosing well-cooked vegetables and opting for soluble fiber sources like oats and bananas, minimizing potential irritants.

2. Lactose Consideration: For those sensitive to lactose, explore lactose-free alternatives or incorporate fermented dairy products like yogurt, which can be better tolerated.

3. Mindful Seasoning: Experiment with gentle herbs and spices to add flavor without overwhelming the digestive system. Avoid excessive use of spicy or highly acidic ingredients.

4. Hydration is Key: Stay well-hydrated to support digestion. Incorporate soups, broths, and herbal teas to maintain fluid balance and ease the digestive process.

5. Smaller, Frequent Meals: Instead of large meals, consider smaller, more frequent meals to prevent overloading the digestive system and provide a steady supply of nutrients.

6. Food Diary: Keep a food diary to track individual responses to different foods, identifying triggers and

aiding in the creation of a personalized, well-tolerated diet.

7. Cooking in Batches: Save time and energy by preparing meals in batches. Store them in portioned containers, ensuring you have readily available, digestive-friendly options.

By incorporating these cooking techniques and tips, individuals with Crohn's disease can enjoy a diverse and flavorful diet while prioritizing digestive well-being. Customizing culinary practices to align with individual preferences and tolerances fosters a positive relationship with food, making the kitchen a source of nourishment and comfort.

Conclusion

Encouragement for Culinary Exploration

Embarking on a culinary exploration is not just about creating meals; it's a journey of discovery, creativity, and self-expression. It's an opportunity to engage with diverse flavors, techniques, and ingredients that can enrich your culinary repertoire and, by extension, your overall well-being. Here's a hearty dose of encouragement for those ready to dive into the world of culinary exploration.

Unlocking Creativity:

Culinary exploration is akin to wielding a paintbrush on a blank canvas. It's a form of artistic expression that allows you to create something unique and deeply personal. As you experiment with flavors, spices, and cooking techniques, you tap into your creativity, discovering new ways to present and savor dishes. The kitchen becomes your creative sanctuary, and every recipe is a chance to showcase your individual style.

Embracing Variety:

The culinary world is a global tapestry woven with an array of ingredients, techniques, and traditions. Embark on a journey that spans continents, exploring the vibrant tapestry of global cuisines. From the aromatic spices of Indian curries to the delicate flavors of Japanese sushi, each culinary tradition offers a new palette to paint your culinary masterpiece. Embrace variety, and let your taste buds travel the world from the comfort of your kitchen.

Building Confidence:

Cooking is a skill that grows with practice, and culinary exploration is your playground. As you experiment with different recipes, you build confidence in the kitchen. Even the simplest tasks, like chopping vegetables or seasoning a dish, contribute to a sense of accomplishment. With each successful creation, your culinary confidence blossoms, encouraging you to take on more complex challenges.

Nourishing Mind and Body:

Culinary exploration isn't just about taste; it's about nourishing your entire being. Engaging with fresh, whole ingredients and crafting balanced, flavorful meals has a profound impact on your physical and mental well-being. You become attuned to the nutritional value of ingredients, making mindful choices that support a healthy lifestyle. The act of cooking itself can be therapeutic, providing a moment of mindfulness in a busy day.

Cultivating Lifelong Learning:

The kitchen is a perpetual classroom where there's always something new to learn. From mastering basic knife skills to delving into the art of fermentation, culinary exploration is a lifelong learning journey. Approach each recipe as an opportunity to expand your culinary knowledge and skills. With the vast array of resources available – cookbooks, online tutorials, and culinary classes – there's no limit to what you can discover.

Connecting with Others:

Culinary exploration is a shared adventure that brings people together. Whether you're cooking for family, friends, or yourself, the act of preparing and sharing a meal fosters connection. It becomes a way to express love, create memories, and bond with others over a shared appreciation for good food.

In the realm of culinary exploration, there are no limits, only endless possibilities waiting to be uncovered. So, tie on that apron, gather your ingredients, and let the delightful aroma of discovery fill your kitchen. Happy cooking!